KEGEL EXERCISES FOR ADULTS

The Essential Guide to Unlock Pelvic Health, Enhance Vitality, and Improve Well-Being with Targeted Techniques

Dr. Theo Leonardo

Made by human

Table of Contents

1 - Introduction

Kegel exercises, also known as pelvic floor exercises, are designed to strengthen the muscles of the pelvic floor. These muscles support the bladder, uterus (in women), and rectum, playing a crucial role in urinary and bowel control, as well as sexual function.

What Are Kegel Exercises?

Kegel exercises involve repeatedly contracting and relaxing the pelvic floor muscles. These exercises can be performed by both men and women and are relatively simple to do. The basic technique involves tightening the muscles that you would use to stop urination, holding the contraction for a few seconds, and then relaxing. This process is repeated several times in a row, multiple times a day.

History and Background

Kegel exercises are named after Dr. Arnold Kegel, an American gynecologist who first described them in 1948. Dr. Kegel developed these exercises as a non-surgical treatment for urinary incontinence in women following childbirth. He published his findings in a study that highlighted the effectiveness of these exercises in improving pelvic muscle strength and reducing incontinence.

Benefits of Kegel Exercises

Improved Bladder Control

Kegel exercises can help both men and women who experience urinary incontinence, a condition where one cannot control urination. Regular practice can strengthen the muscles that control the bladder, reducing or eliminating episodes of leakage.

Enhanced Sexual Function

Strengthening the pelvic floor muscles can lead to increased sexual sensation and improved sexual performance. In women, stronger pelvic floor muscles can lead to enhanced arousal, orgasm, and overall sexual satisfaction. In men, these exercises can help with erectile function and ejaculation control.

Support During Pregnancy and Postpartum Recovery

For women, doing Kegel exercises during pregnancy can help prepare the pelvic floor muscles for the stresses of childbirth. Postpartum, these exercises can aid in recovery by improving muscle tone and reducing the risk of postpartum urinary incontinence.

Prevention of Pelvic Organ Prolapse

Regular Kegel exercises can help prevent pelvic organ prolapse, a condition where the pelvic organs drop from their normal position due to weakened pelvic floor muscles. This is particularly important for women as they age or after childbirth.

Bowel Control

Kegel exercises can also benefit those who suffer from fecal incontinence by strengthening the muscles that control bowel movements.

Post-Surgical Recovery

For men, Kegel exercises are often recommended after prostate surgery to help regain urinary control and improve sexual function.

Kegel exercises are a simple, non-invasive way to strengthen the pelvic floor muscles, offering a range of benefits for both men and women across various stages of life.

2 - Anatomy and Physiology

Understanding the Pelvic Floor Muscles

The pelvic floor muscles are a group of muscles and connective tissues that span the base of the pelvis. They support the pelvic organs, which include the bladder, intestines, and uterus (in women). The key muscles of the pelvic floor include:

1. Levator Ani: This is the largest component, consisting

of three parts – the pubococcygeus, puborectalis, and iliococcygeus muscles. It plays a crucial role in maintaining continence and supporting pelvic organs.

2. Coccygeus: This muscle supports the pelvic organs and stabilizes the coccyx (tailbone).

3. Bulbospongiosus: In men, this muscle helps with erections and ejaculation, while in women, it constricts the vaginal orifice.

4. Ischiocavernosus: This muscle helps maintain erections in men and tenses the vagina in women.

5. Transverse Perineal Muscles: These provide support to the pelvic floor.

The pelvic floor muscles work together with the abdominal and back muscles to stabilize and support the spine and pelvis.

How Kegels Affect the Body

Kegel exercises specifically target the pelvic floor muscles, leading to several physiological benefits:

1. Increased Muscle Strength and Tone: Regular Kegel exercises strengthen the pelvic floor muscles, improving their ability to support pelvic organs and maintain continence.

2. Improved Blood Flow: Like other muscles, the pelvic floor muscles benefit from

increased blood flow during exercise. Improved circulation can enhance tissue health and function.

3. Enhanced Neural Control: Repeatedly contracting and relaxing the pelvic floor muscles can improve neuromuscular control, making it easier to engage these muscles when needed.

4. Support for Pelvic Organs: Strengthening these muscles provides better support for the bladder, intestines, and uterus, reducing the risk of

prolapse and other pelvic organ dysfunctions.

5. Improved Bladder and Bowel Control: By strengthening the muscles that control the urethra and anus, Kegel exercises can reduce episodes of urinary and fecal incontinence.

6. Sexual Health Benefits: For both men and women, stronger pelvic floor muscles can enhance sexual pleasure and function. In men, they can help with erections and ejaculation control, while in women, they can increase

vaginal tone and orgasm intensity.

7. Post-Surgical Recovery: After surgeries like prostatectomy in men or childbirth in women, Kegel exercises can help restore muscle strength and function.

Kegel exercises contribute to better pelvic health, improved quality of life, and enhanced physical and sexual function by directly impacting the strength and coordination of the pelvic floor muscles.

3 - Getting Started

Identifying the Right Muscles

Before starting Kegel exercises, it is essential to identify the correct muscles. Here are a few methods to help locate the pelvic floor muscles:

1. Stopping the Flow of Urine: One of the simplest ways to identify the pelvic floor muscles is by attempting to stop the flow of urine midstream. The muscles you

use to achieve this are your pelvic floor muscles. However, this method should only be used for identification purposes and not as a regular exercise practice.

2. Sensation of Lifting: Imagine you are trying to lift a small marble with your vaginal muscles (for women) or pulling your penis inward (for men). The muscles you engage in this process are your pelvic floor muscles.

3. Mirror Method: For women, using a mirror to observe the perineal area while attempting

to contract the pelvic floor muscles can help visualize the lifting of the pelvic floor.

4. Finger Method: Insert a clean finger into the vagina (for women) or anus (for men) and try to squeeze the muscles around the finger. If you feel a tightening around the finger, you are using the correct muscles.

Proper Technique for Performing Kegels

Once you've identified the pelvic floor muscles, follow

these steps to perform Kegel exercises correctly:

1. Find a Comfortable Position: You can do Kegel exercises while sitting, lying down, or standing. Choose a position where you can comfortably relax.

2. Contract the Muscles: Tighten the pelvic floor muscles, lifting them upwards. Hold this contraction for about 3 to 5 seconds.

3. Relax the Muscles: Release the contraction and relax the muscles completely for an

equal amount of time (3 to 5 seconds).

4. Repeat: Perform 10 to 15 repetitions in one session. Aim to do three sessions per day.

5. Gradual Increase: As your muscles get stronger, gradually increase the duration of each contraction and relaxation, working up to 10 seconds each.

Common Mistakes to Avoid

1. Using the Wrong Muscles: Ensure you are only using your pelvic floor muscles.

Avoid tightening your abdomen, thighs, or buttocks.

2. Holding Your Breath: Breathe normally throughout the exercise. Holding your breath can create unnecessary tension in your body.

3. Overdoing It: More isn't always better. Over-exercising the pelvic floor muscles can lead to muscle fatigue and potential strain. Stick to the recommended number of repetitions and sets.

4. Incomplete Relaxation: Make sure to fully relax the pelvic floor muscles between contractions. This ensures the muscles do not remain in a constant state of tension.

5. Inconsistent Practice: Consistency is key. Try to incorporate Kegel exercises into your daily routine to achieve the best results. Set reminders or link them to other daily activities like brushing your teeth.

By correctly identifying the pelvic floor muscles and practicing the proper technique, you can effectively perform Kegel exercises and enjoy their numerous benefits.

4 - Kegel Exercises for Different Populations

Kegels for Women

During Pregnancy

Benefits:

- Strengthens pelvic floor muscles to support the growing baby.

- Helps prevent urinary incontinence during and after pregnancy.

- Prepares the muscles for the stress of childbirth, potentially reducing labor time and complications.

Tips:

- Begin practicing Kegel exercises early in pregnancy.

- Perform Kegels while sitting, standing, or lying down to find the most comfortable position.

- Aim for 10-15 repetitions, three times a day.

Postpartum

Benefits:

- Aids in recovery of pelvic floor muscles stretched or weakened during childbirth.

- Reduces the risk of postpartum urinary incontinence.

- Helps with healing episiotomies or perineal tears by improving blood flow.

Tips:

- Start Kegel exercises as soon as you feel comfortable after delivery, usually a few days postpartum.

- Begin with gentle contractions and gradually increase intensity and duration.

- Incorporate Kegels into daily routines, such as feeding the baby or during diaper changes.

Menopause

Benefits:

- Helps counteract the weakening of pelvic floor muscles due to decreased estrogen levels.

- Reduces the risk of urinary incontinence and pelvic organ prolapse.

- Improves sexual function and sensation.

Tips:

- Consistency is key; make Kegel exercises a part of your daily routine.

- Use biofeedback devices or vaginal weights for additional

resistance and better muscle awareness.

- Combine Kegel exercises with hormone replacement therapy (if prescribed) for optimal results.

Kegels for Men

Prostate Health

Benefits:

- Strengthens pelvic floor muscles, aiding in urinary control post-prostate surgery.

- Reduces symptoms of benign prostatic hyperplasia

(BPH) by improving bladder control.

- Helps manage chronic prostatitis symptoms by reducing pelvic pain and discomfort.

Tips:

- Start Kegel exercises before prostate surgery to build muscle strength.

- Post-surgery, begin with gentle contractions and gradually increase intensity.

- Perform exercises regularly, aiming for 10-15 repetitions, three times a day.

Erectile Dysfunction

Benefits:

- Improves blood flow to the pelvic region, enhancing erectile function.

- Strengthens the muscles involved in erection and ejaculation.

- Boosts confidence and sexual performance.

Tips:

- Identify the correct muscles by stopping the flow of urine or imagining pulling the penis inward.

- Start with shorter holds (3-5 seconds) and gradually increase to longer holds (10 seconds).

- Be patient and consistent, as improvements may take several weeks to become noticeable.

General Tips for All Populations

1.   Stay Consistent: Incorporate Kegel exercises into your daily routine for the best results.

2.   Monitor Progress: Keep track of your progress and gradually increase the intensity and duration of exercises as your muscles strengthen.

3.   Seek Professional Guidance: If you are unsure about your technique or need personalized advice, consult a

healthcare provider or pelvic floor therapist.

4. Avoid Straining: Ensure you are not overexerting yourself. Kegel exercises should not cause pain or discomfort.

5. Combine with Other Exercises: Complement Kegel exercises with other core-strengthening activities like Pilates or yoga for overall pelvic health.

By tailoring Kegel exercises to specific populations, individuals can address their unique needs and achieve better pelvic health outcomes.

5 - Advanced Kegel Techniques

Variations and Progressions

As you become more comfortable with basic Kegel exercises, you can introduce variations and progressions to further challenge and strengthen your pelvic floor muscles.

1. Elevator Kegels:

- Imagine your pelvic floor muscles as an elevator. Slowly lift the muscles to the first floor (slight contraction), hold for a second, then lift to the second floor (stronger contraction), and so on until you reach the top floor (maximum contraction). Reverse the process on the way down.

- This exercise helps with muscle control and endurance.

2. Quick Flicks:

- Quickly contract and release the pelvic floor muscles. Perform 10 rapid contractions followed by a rest period.

   - This variation helps improve the speed and responsiveness of the muscles.

3. Reverse Kegels:

   - Focus on relaxing and gently pushing the pelvic floor muscles downward, as if trying to push something out.

   - This technique can help balance the contraction and relaxation phases and improve overall muscle control.

4. Bridge with Kegels:

- Lie on your back with knees bent and feet flat on the floor. Lift your hips into a bridge position while simultaneously performing a Kegel contraction. Hold for a few seconds, then lower your hips and relax the muscles.

- This exercise combines core and pelvic floor strengthening.

Integrating Kegels with Other Exercises

Incorporating Kegel exercises into your regular workout routine can enhance overall pelvic health and fitness.

1. Pilates:

- Many Pilates exercises naturally engage the pelvic floor. Focus on performing Kegels during exercises like the pelvic tilt, leg lifts, and the hundred.

2. Yoga:

-       Integrate   Kegel contractions during poses such as the bridge pose (Setu Bandhasana), child's pose (Balasana), and cat-cow pose (Marjaryasana-Bitilasana).

3. Strength Training:

- Perform Kegels during weightlifting exercises such as squats, deadlifts, and lunges. Engage the pelvic floor muscles at the same time as your core to enhance stability and control.

4. Cardio:

- Practice Kegels while walking, running, or cycling by rhythmically contracting and relaxing the pelvic floor muscles.

Tools and Devices to Enhance Results

Several tools and devices can help you get the most out of your Kegel exercises by providing resistance, feedback, or guidance.

1. Kegel Balls or Ben Wa Balls:

- Insert these weighted balls into the vagina. The added weight provides resistance, making your pelvic floor muscles work harder to hold them in place.

2. Biofeedback Devices:

- These devices use sensors to measure the strength of your pelvic floor contractions and provide real-time feedback. They can help ensure you are performing the exercises correctly and track your progress over time.

3.   Electrical   Stimulation Devices:

- These devices deliver small electrical pulses to the pelvic floor muscles, causing them to contract. They can be especially helpful for individuals with weak pelvic muscles or difficulty performing Kegels independently.

4. Smartphone Apps:

- Several apps are available that provide guided Kegel

exercise routines, reminders, and progress tracking. Examples include Elvie, Kegel Trainer, and Perifit.

5. Resistance Trainers:

- Devices like the Elvie Trainer and kGoal provide resistance and real-time feedback via a connected app, making exercises more engaging and effective.

By incorporating advanced techniques, integrating Kegels with other exercises, and using specialized tools and devices, you can enhance the

effectiveness of your pelvic
floor training and achieve
better results.

6 - Creating a Routine

How Often to Do Kegels

For optimal results, consistency and frequency are key when performing Kegel exercises. Here's a general guideline:

1. Daily Practice: Aim to perform Kegel exercises daily. Establishing a routine ensures you don't skip sessions.

2. Frequency: Start with three sets of 10-15 repetitions each day. Gradually increase the number of sets as your pelvic

floor muscles become stronger.

3. Duration: Hold each contraction for 3-5 seconds initially, and then relax for the same amount of time. As you progress, increase the hold duration to 10 seconds.

Building a Sustainable Practice

1. Set Reminders: Use alarms, smartphone apps, or sticky notes to remind you to perform your Kegel exercises throughout the day.

2. Link to Daily Activities: Incorporate Kegel exercises into your routine by linking them to daily activities such as brushing your teeth, commuting, or watching TV.

3. Stay Comfortable: Perform Kegel exercises in various positions (sitting, standing, lying down) to find what's most comfortable for you.

4. Gradual Progression: Start with shorter hold times and fewer repetitions. Gradually increase the intensity, duration, and number of

repetitions as your muscles strengthen.

5. Mindfulness and Focus: Pay close attention to your body and ensure you are using the correct muscles. Avoid tensing other muscle groups like the abdomen, buttocks, or thighs.

6. Stay Motivated: Track your progress and celebrate small milestones to stay motivated. Understand that results may take a few weeks to become noticeable.

Tracking Progress and Results

1. Set Clear Goals: Define what you want to achieve with your Kegel exercises, whether it's improved bladder control, enhanced sexual function, or overall pelvic health.

2. Keep a Journal: Maintain a log of your Kegel exercises, noting the date, time, duration of contractions, and number of repetitions. This will help you track consistency and progress over time.

3. Use Apps and Devices: Leverage technology such as smartphone apps or biofeedback devices to monitor your progress. These tools can provide real-time feedback and track improvements in muscle strength and endurance.

4. Monitor Symptoms: Pay attention to any changes in your symptoms, such as reduced urinary incontinence, less pelvic discomfort, or improved sexual function. Note these changes in your journal.

5. Regular Check-ins: Set periodic check-ins with a healthcare provider or pelvic floor therapist to assess your progress and make any necessary adjustments to your routine.

6. Adjust Routine as Needed: Based on your progress and feedback, adjust your routine to include more advanced exercises, increase the number of repetitions, or incorporate additional tools and devices.

By following a consistent routine, gradually increasing

the intensity, and tracking your progress, you can build a sustainable Kegel exercise practice that effectively strengthens your pelvic floor muscles and enhances your overall pelvic health.

7 - Troubleshooting and FAQs

Common Issues and Solutions

1. Difficulty Identifying the Right Muscles

- Issue: Struggling to isolate the pelvic floor muscles.

- Solution: Try different methods to identify the muscles, such as stopping the flow of urine midstream or inserting a clean finger and contracting around it. Consult a pelvic floor therapist for personalized guidance.

2. Straining or Overexerting

- Issue: Experiencing discomfort or pain while doing Kegel exercises.

- Solution: Ensure you are not tensing other muscle groups (e.g., abdomen, thighs, or buttocks). Start with shorter holds and fewer repetitions, and gradually increase as your muscles strengthen.

3. Inconsistent Results

- Issue: Not seeing improvements despite regular practice.

- Solution: Check your technique to ensure proper muscle engagement. Keep track of your progress and make adjustments to your routine if needed. It can take several weeks to notice significant changes.

4. Difficulty Relaxing the Muscles

- Issue: Finding it hard to fully relax the pelvic floor muscles between contractions.

- Solution: Focus on consciously relaxing the muscles after each contraction. Practice deep breathing exercises to help with relaxation.

5. Bladder or Bowel Discomfort

- Issue: Experiencing discomfort in the bladder or

bowel during or after Kegel exercises.

- Solution: Ensure you are using the correct muscles and not overexerting yourself. If discomfort persists, consult a healthcare provider to rule out any underlying issues.

6. Forgetfulness or Lack of Motivation

- Issue: Forgetting to do Kegel exercises or struggling to stay motivated.

- Solution: Set reminders, link exercises to daily activities, or use apps to stay on track. Setting small, achievable goals can also help maintain motivation.

When to Seek Professional Help

1. Persistent Pain or Discomfort

   - When to Seek Help: If you experience ongoing pain or discomfort during or after Kegel exercises.

   - Professional Help: Consult a healthcare provider or a pelvic floor therapist to identify the cause and receive appropriate treatment.

2. Inability to Identify Pelvic Floor Muscles

   - When to Seek Help: If you have trouble identifying and isolating the pelvic floor muscles despite trying various methods.

   - Professional Help: A pelvic floor therapist can provide guidance and exercises to help you correctly engage these muscles.

3. Severe Urinary or Fecal Incontinence

- When to Seek Help: If you experience severe or worsening urinary or fecal incontinence despite regular Kegel practice.

- Professional Help: Consult a urologist or gastroenterologist for a comprehensive evaluation and treatment options.

4. Prolonged Lack of Improvement

- When to Seek Help: If you do not notice any improvements in your symptoms after several weeks of consistent practice.

   -   Professional Help: A healthcare provider or pelvic floor therapist can assess your technique and make necessary adjustments to your routine.

5. Post-Surgical Complications

   - When to Seek Help: After surgeries such as prostatectomy or childbirth, if you experience complications or difficulties with recovery.

   - Professional Help: Consult your surgeon or a pelvic floor

therapist for a tailored rehabilitation plan and guidance on resuming Kegel exercises.

6. Pelvic Pain or Discomfort

   - When to Seek Help: If you experience persistent pelvic pain or discomfort unrelated to Kegel exercises.

   - Professional Help: A healthcare provider can evaluate for conditions like pelvic inflammatory disease or pelvic floor dysfunction.

By addressing common issues and knowing when to seek

professional help, you can effectively manage and troubleshoot any challenges with Kegel exercises, ensuring a successful and beneficial practice.

8 - Lifestyle and Kegel Exercises

Nutrition and Hydration

1. Nutrition:

- Balanced Diet: A diet rich in fruits, vegetables, whole grains, lean proteins, and healthy fats supports overall health, including pelvic health. Nutrients like fiber can help prevent constipation, which reduces strain on the pelvic floor.

- Avoid Irritants: Limit intake of caffeine, alcohol,

and spicy foods, which can irritate the bladder and exacerbate urinary symptoms.

-       Healthy   Weight: Maintaining a healthy weight helps reduce pressure on the pelvic floor muscles, thereby supporting better function and reducing the risk of incontinence and prolapse.

2. Hydration:

- Adequate Fluid Intake: Drink plenty of water throughout the day to stay hydrated. Proper hydration supports overall bodily functions, including bladder health.

- Balanced Consumption: While it's important to stay hydrated, avoid excessive fluid intake right before bed to minimize nighttime bathroom trips.

Stress Management

1. Impact on Pelvic Floor Health:

- Stress and Tension: Chronic stress can lead to muscle tension, including in the pelvic floor, which may affect Kegel exercise effectiveness and overall pelvic health.

- Emotional Well-being: Stress can exacerbate symptoms like urinary incontinence and pelvic pain. Managing stress can improve your overall quality of life and pelvic health.

2. Techniques for Stress Management:

- Mindfulness and Meditation: Practicing mindfulness and meditation can help reduce stress and promote relaxation, benefiting both your mental and pelvic health.

- Deep Breathing Exercises: Incorporate deep breathing exercises into your daily routine to help manage stress and promote relaxation.

- Regular Physical Activity: Engage in regular exercise, such as walking, swimming, or yoga, to reduce stress and support overall well-being.

- Adequate Sleep: Ensure you get enough restful sleep each night to help manage stress and support bodily functions, including muscle recovery and pelvic health.

Overall Pelvic Health

1. Exercise Variety:

   - Strengthening Exercises: In addition to Kegels, include other exercises that strengthen the core, hips, and lower back. This helps provide additional support to the pelvic floor.

   - Flexibility and Mobility: Incorporate stretching and flexibility exercises to maintain pelvic mobility and prevent stiffness.

2. Posture and Body Mechanics:

- Proper Posture: Maintain good posture to avoid unnecessary pressure on the pelvic floor. Sitting and standing with proper alignment helps reduce strain on pelvic muscles.

- Safe Lifting Techniques: Use correct lifting techniques, such as bending at the knees rather than the waist, to avoid putting excessive pressure on the pelvic floor.

3. Regular Health Check-ups:

- Routine Exams: Regular check-ups with your healthcare provider can help monitor pelvic health and address any concerns or symptoms early.

- Pelvic Floor Therapy: If you experience persistent issues, consider consulting a pelvic floor therapist for personalized advice and treatments.

4. Healthy Habits:

- Avoid Smoking: Smoking can contribute to pelvic floor

problems and other health issues. Quitting smoking supports overall pelvic health and reduces the risk of complications.

- Balanced Lifestyle: A well-rounded lifestyle that includes a healthy diet, regular exercise, and stress management supports optimal pelvic floor function and overall health.

By integrating these lifestyle factors with your Kegel exercise routine, you can enhance the effectiveness of your pelvic floor training and

support overall pelvic health
and well-being.

THE END

www.ingramcontent.com/pod-product-compliance
Lightning Source LLC
Chambersburg PA
CBHW050831250726
48653CB00006B/2543